T0033451

MINDFUL
MICRODOSING
A Guidebook and Journal

MINDFUL MICRODOSING
A Guidebook and Journal

by

LAUREN ALDERFER

illustrations by

MARIANA JUAREZ

GREEN WRITERS PRESS
Brattleboro, Vermont

Copyright © 2024 by Lauren Alderfer, Ph.D.

All rights reserved. No part of this book may be reproduced in any manner without written permission except in the case of brief quotations included in critical articles and reviews.

The publisher and the author are providing this book and its contents on an "as is" basis and make no representations or warranties of any kind with respect to this book or its contents. The publisher and the author disclaim all such representations and warranties, including but not limited to warranties of healthcare for a particular purpose. In addition, the publisher and the author assume no responsibility for errors, inaccuracies, omissions, or any other inconsistencies herein. The content of this book is for entertainment and informational purposes only and is not intended to diagnose, treat, cure, or prevent any condition or disease. You understand that this book is not intended as a substitute for consultation with a licensed practitioner. Please consult with your own physician or healthcare specialist regarding the suggestions and recommendations made in this book. Reading and/or using this book implies your acceptance of this disclaimer.

Printed in the United States.

10 9 8 7 6 5 4 3 2 1

Green Writers Press is a Vermont-based publisher whose mission is to spread a message of hope and renewal through the words and images we publish. Throughout, we will adhere to our commitment to preserving and protecting the natural resources of the earth. To that end, a percentage of our proceeds will be donated to environmental and social-activist groups. Green Writers Press gratefully acknowledges support from individual donors, friends, and readers to help support the environment and our publishing initiative.

Green
writers
press

Giving Voice to Writers & Artists Who Will Make the World a Better Place
Green Writers Press | Brattleboro, Vermont
www.greenwriterspress.com

ISBN: 979-8-9876631-3-4

COVER ART/DESIGN:
Mariana Juarez/Hannah Alderfer

For more information, visit the author's website:
www.laurenalderfer.com

PRINTED ON 30% POST-CONSUMER FIBER WITH STOCK SHEETS THAT ARE FOREST STEWARDSHIP COUNCIL® (FSC®) CERTIFIED THAT COME FROM MANAGED FORESTS THAT GUARANTEE RESPONSIBLE ENVIRONMENTAL, SOCIAL, AND ECONOMIC PRACTICES. PRINTED BY SHERIDAN PRINTERS.

A hallmark of mindfulness is the silencing of the mind,
giving way to the expanding expression of the heart in the
all-knowing present moment. In that stillness there emerges
a sacred connection to all. Mindful microdosing cultivates this
spaciousness of mind and expansiveness of heart.

CONTENTS

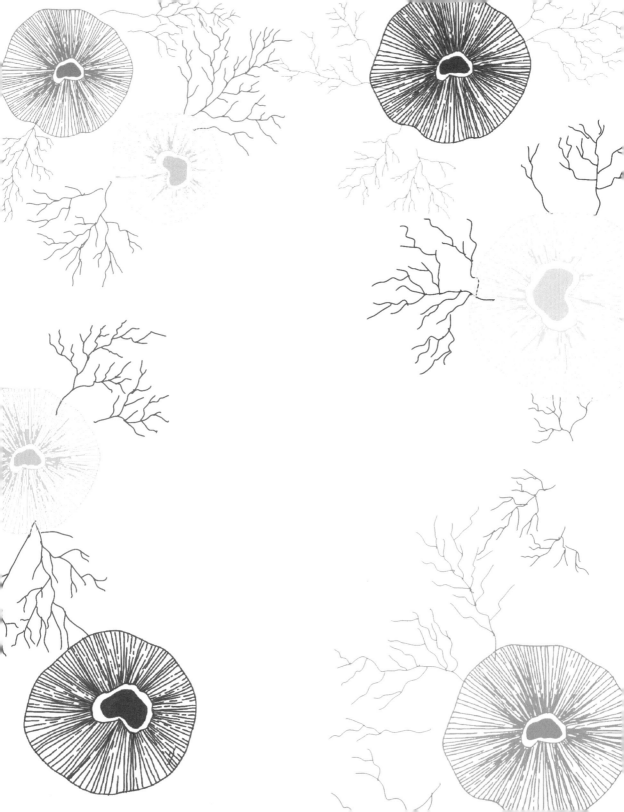

ELCOME TO *Mindful Microdosing: A Guidebook and Journal*. May it serve you as you embark on your own unique journey. What follows are invitations, invitations to weave together mindfulness and microdosing. It supports direct experience and self-reflection to encourage an ever-evolving, spiraling process of experiential learning, growing awareness, and self-discovery. This book is born out of this seed of understanding. Both mindfulness and psychedelics offer a gateway to touch the wonder of your essential nature, one based on deep wisdom that springs from a oneness in expanding love. The guidebook and journal offer a foundation for your journey; for how you approach it can be the crucial key that opens the gateway to your inner garden. The harvest of what will be sown germinates and reveals itself in full light. This book invites ways to continually integrate your experience and cultivate such a garden and nourish its growth.

Microdosing in the natural world has had a historical trajectory that has now found its way into the lives of millions around the globe. Microdosing synthetic substances such as LSD and MDMA are being researched and found to have therapeutic value. Traditional substances, entheogenic plants, and fungi being researched and used for microdosing include psilocybin mushrooms, ayahuasca (and one of its non-psychoactive vines, known as Whole B. Caapi), huachuma (also known as San Pedro cactus); and surprisingly, even cannabis. Ingesting psilocybin from mushrooms is one of the most common ways to microdose. Therefore mushrooms, understood as sacred earth medicine, find their presence throughout the book in an illustrative and metaphorical form. If you do choose another substance, the book's mindfulness-based approach is equally applicable to your experience. The first section takes a look at mindfulness, microdosing, the guidebook, and journaling. In this section, you will find questions, posed as queries for self-reflection, sprinkled throughout. You may prefer to skip over these questions or return to them when the time feels right. Similarly, you may want to skip ahead to immerse yourself in areas of focus that speak to you. The second section is for journaling. It is divided into three areas of focus: Preparation, Journey, and Integration. Each of these sections begins with an intricate drawing for you to color in if you choose. Coloring in these playful illustrations may calm the mind and alight the heart to support a more mindful experience. After each illustration, there are journaling pages with faint or more noticeable imagery with the invitation for your heart and mind to lead the way in however you decide to co-create your journal. The last section sets the ground for safe exploration with some charts and mindful inquiries for your consideration. So let the journal be your friend and ally, lending support and a safe container as you cultivate your path to optimal well-being and greater wholeness.

Let us honor wisdom keepers of all lands and traditions past, present, and future, as well as the generosity of the sacred earth medicines and all sentient beings. I also want to express deep gratitude for connecting to you, the reader, over time and place through the offering and spirit of *Mindful Microdosing: A Guidebook and Journal*.

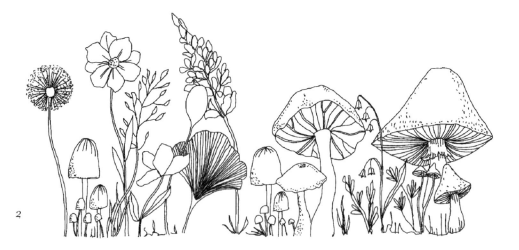

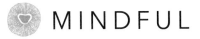 # MINDFUL

Many long-time mindfulness practitioners have found that a micro or macro experience affirms their many years of dedicated effort to cultivate mindfulness. Conversely, many people find these sacred psychedelic experiences lead them to practice mindfulness for the first time in their lives. Microdosing in a mindful way is complementary to both mindfulness and microdosing—it invites in the possibility of an embodied experience of expanding wisdom and compassion in the interconnected web of life. It can open the door beyond the linear, individualized "I" to a sense of growing heartfelt connection to something greater. When you embody this connection, imbued with ever-expanding love and peace, you walk in this world more lightly.

His Holiness the XIV Dalai Lama speaks of mindfulness as an "…inner peace of an alert and calm mind," and that it is the source of real happiness and good health. "Mindfulness is a pause, the space between stimulus and response: where choice is made," according to mindfulness teacher Tara Brach. The translation of mindfulness from the original Pali, *sati*, includes awareness, to remember, and to recollect. Indeed, mindfulness leads you home to be aware of and to remember and recollect your own true nature of abiding peace and love. It asks you to live in this wholeness just as you are. Mindfulness, according to Thich Nhat Hanh, a Vietnamese Zen Buddhist monk, ". . . is to become completely alive and live deeply each moment of your daily life. Mindfulness helps you touch the wonders of life for self-nourishment and healing."

Being mindful, above all else, is heart-centered. This book was designed so that both your heart and mind can be revealed with growing clarity. When you calm the monkey mind of its busy doing it invites in simply being. Then the light of mindful awareness and the expanding expression of the heart shine more brightly in the present moment. Thus, to be mindful is an essential ingredient in *Mindful Microdosing: A Guidebook and Journal*. Practicing mindfulness helps wisdom and compassion weave their way through these pages and into your experience; it enhances and helps determine the very nature of your unfolding journey.

There are a plethora of mindfulness practices, such as observing the natural breath with equanimity and without changing a thing, scanning your body to observe sensations, and focusing on an object and gently bringing your mind back to that focus without judgment. These are some commonly practiced techniques, and there are so many other forms of mind training. The cornerstone of most mindfulness practices is the skillful means to bring awareness, without judgment, to what you observe. Rather than being reactive, there is growing awareness that naturally leads to better self-regulation of emotions. Simply holding the light of awareness with a neutral but loving understanding offers a most essential tool when ingesting psychedelics: to be aware of what arises from a place of calm abiding.

Beginning your unique journey in a mindful way invites you to deeply honor all that has arisen to make this present moment possible, to all that led up to it, and to all that may benefit from it now and in the future. This is an opportunity to to acknowledge and express an outpouring of gratitude to wisdom keepers past, present, and future, to the plant and animal worlds and their innate wisdom, indeed to all of nature, and to all sentient beings. You are invited to close your eyes and bring awareness to deep within your belly. Feel your belly rise and expand on the inhalation, and observe it gently sink back in on the exhalation. Continue to take a few more mindful breaths, calming both body and mind, to contemplate this moment.

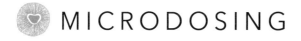

MICRODOSING

Microdosing is not a pill to be taken like an aspirin to get rid of a headache. Instead, it offers the possibility to connect and live in a greater presence of being. Microdosing supports overall health and well-being, and in so doing, the headache may very well disappear. Microdosing can be understood as a harmonious interplay with the natural world through the reverent use of earth and plant medicine. This is similar to the understanding behind Traditional Chinese Medicine, Ayurveda, Tibetan medicine, homeopathy, and integrative medicine, to name just a few similar examples.

Mushroom foraging has been carried out all over the world through the ages to this day. Credit and honor is given to the Mazatec *curandera* María Sabina of Oaxaca, Mexico for her wisdom and compassion and the pivotal role she played, including great sacrifice, in the intertwining history of how magic mushrooms reached the USA and into the hands of millions today. Though there is much focus on macrodosing, two leading figures in today's burgeoning microdosing landscape are Dr. James Fadiman and Paul Stamets; in fact, there are two main microdosing protocols named after them. According to Stamets microdosing is non-intoxicating, and Dr. Fadiman says, "Microdosing is not sub-perceptual, but it is below the threshold without psychedelic effects; it is not without observable effects." You may appreciate a daisy in full bloom more than usual, and see its colors more brilliantly than you normally do, but the flower is not changing shape or speaking to you. If it does, you are not microdosing!

Microdosing promotes the formation of neural connections, increasing the brain's neuroplasticity. This can show up in a variety of ways; for example, a greater sense of grounding, ease, focus, creativity, and mental clarity. You may feel more enthusiasm, motivation, social ability, or empathy for others. Indeed, microdosing alights deeper networks in both your inner and outer worlds. You may find yourself out in nature more, or that nature's wisdom is showing up in ways new to you. In whatever way you feel this interconnection, there is an invitation to embody "…a mutual flourishing," as Robin Wall Kimmerer, member of the Citizen Potawatomi Nation, botanist, and professor writes of the reciprocal relationship in which you are both beneficiary and giver.. This reciprocal relationship, especially if it is unfamiliar to you, can be a like a Tibetan *terma*, a hidden treasure that reveals itself at the right time in its own way.

Indigenous peoples, indeed peoples of all traditions, have over centuries reverently intertwined their ways of being with the natural world. They live with heart and mind in connection to, not separate from, listening and responding to the wise, living intelligence they know to be inherent in nature. Mushrooms exhibit DNA that is more than one billion years old. Classified as fungi, their DNA is more similar to humans than to plants. How mind-boggling and inspiring! Fifth-generation medicine woman Xochitl Ashe reminds us that, "…sacred plant medicine is ancestral medicine." What ancestral wisdom is alive in you? What reciprocal relationship has been born? What mutual flourishing may come into being?

Spores are the powdery puffballs that germinate into mushrooms. Both mushrooms and their spores expand at a phenomenal rate. Inspired by indigenous ways of understanding, you can look at the expansive nature of mushrooms, beginning with their spores, and ask yourself how it may inform you. You may consider contemplating how this same expansive nature may be revealed in you: in your brain, daily life, and relationship with the natural world.

After dispersing in the sky, spores usually find their way to the ground, recreating, transforming, and beginning to form new connections. They grow in networks, with nodes forming so that new networks grow in all directions: the possibilities limitless. Can you also hold the belief that you have infinite possibilities? That anything is possible? Belief and hope, like the mycelial network, connected fungal threads born out of spores, are unseen, but they hold great force behind anything undertaken in life. This underground mycelial network of intelligence, creating extensive pathways, is one of the fastest growing organisms alive. Can you make room for a similar miraculous unfolding?

Above ground, spores burst into their fruit: the mushroom. How are you coming into your own full expression? A mushroom's resilience is remarkable. Though relatively light in weight, a mushroom has the strength to both sway to the force of the wind and stand its ground. Can you feel your strength while remaining open-hearted? Mushrooms can heal but they can also kill. Do your thoughts, words, and deeds support healing, or do they carry poison? What habits of mind and daily choices might be unhealthy ones? What do you choose that nourishes wholeness and optimizes well-being?

A mushroom's life cycle includes its natural decomposition. Decay is an inevitable transformation present throughout the living world. How do you approach different stages of your own life? Do you live with the understanding of your own impermanence and the impermanent nature of all life? The beauty in the mushroom's decay is that it provides needed nutrients for the cycle to continue. What are some of the gifts you leave for others?

The mushroom's journey offers guideposts for your own garden of life. I invite you to approach microdosing with this understanding. Or at the very least, see if you can remain open to the living intelligence inherent in mushrooms expressing itself in you in wise and loving ways. If you can greet and receive its spirit with this possibility, you are entering into what is understood as right relationship. As psychedelics scientist Katherine MacLean explains, experiences with mushrooms are all about relationship. This is a deeply meaningful and transformational way of microdosing: reverently receiving the mushrooms as friend, ally, teacher, and companion.

GUIDEBOOK & JOURNAL

Detailed descriptions of each section of the journal serve as a guidebook for your mindful microdosing process. They offer a common way to approach, experience, and feel the impact of microdosing. These three sections—Preparation, Journey, and Integration—are presented in succession on the following pages, but they are, in fact, a spiraling, intertwining cycle of all three. You may go in order but then find yourself adding more to previous sections. Much like the double helix of your DNA and that of mushrooms, the process, rather than being linear, is one of living movement, of self-evolving, ongoing creation. This creation is playful in nature, and so *Mindful Microdosing: A Guidebook and Journal* invites your own playfulness and fun to express themselves on its pages. In the Journal section, enjoy coloring in the illustrations, draw additions of your own, doodle and create with a sense of childlike abandon. Some of the mushrooms, in Spanish, are called little children, *los niñitos*. Let your inner child free! Connect to its nature and let it express itself through you!

Preparation — Set and Setting

The first section is the preparation for what lies ahead. When gardening, you would first purview the land, find a patch, and assess its soil. You might daydream about your garden for days, weeks, or months before actually choosing which spot. You would decide what to grow, and visualize what your garden would look like. A mindful microdosing journey begins in this same spirit. Like contemplating your garden, you prepare the soil of your heart and mind as part of, or even prior to, preparation. Then, with some tending, you observe what you planted and watch what grows. Eventually you reap the fruit of your efforts, and with a thankful heart, you break bread and share the harvest with others. This same invitation is present throughout *Mindful Microdosing: A Guidebook and Journal*.

Set typically refers to your mindset. Setting generally refers to your physical and social environment. What are some of your expectations? How are you feeling? How supportive are your physical surroundings? What considerations have you made for the day's activities? For silence or music? What of your outdoor environment? Friends you'll be with? Far more subtle and elaborate factors can be part of set and setting, but most importantly, you can approach set and setting with greater mindfulness by making choices with discernment and intentionality. Sourcing your substance, its reliability, and the proper dose are also very important factors. The more knowledge you have about your choices, combined with the safest set and setting, give you greater agency in preparing for your journey. This kind of mindful consumption, along with a frame of mind filled with a spaciousness of calm and ease, better welcomes whatever arises to enhance your journey.

When you actively microdose, an environment that optimizes the experience is ideal. Use of recreational substances detract, as does frenetic activity. Nourishing activities such as being outdoors in nature, breathwork, or any mindfulness practice that increases a sense of calm abiding and centering is encouraged. You may want to jot some of your nourishing activities down, as well as some of your detractors. This can serve as a reminder, ensuring your setting for the journey stays at its best.

Self-assessing to get a baseline as a starting point is commonly done as part of preparation. This might be done in a more traditional way by using a framework or lens to look at specific factors that you want to track before, during, and after your journey. If you decide to use a specific paradigm to get a baseline, then you should note your findings in this Preparation section. However, you will find a more detailed discussion and presentation of some of these frameworks in the next section: Journey - Active Microdosing.

You may also give self-expression to where you are at this moment in more non-linear ways. This may take the form of free flow writing; drawing a body map and coloring inside the outline to illustrate your embodied experiences and perceptions; a life-line to write out or illustrate events that chronicle your life; or a sketch or collage. This is your place to doodle, write, draw, and create whatever feels right for you. This is your garden. It may have some weeds, or even parts completely overgrown with weeds. If so, add to the drawing of the garden found on the first page of this section or create a garden of your own that best portrays your own fertile ground. Let this section flourish with an outpouring that reflects a mirror to the garden of your life.

Preparation now turns to a more inward element. It is here where the connection to your deepest intention comes to the surface. It is this intention that is an essential part of making a mindful microdosing journey mindful. It may take days or even weeks to discover, but it is your intention that becomes the breath of life connecting, traveling through, and guiding your experience.

The concept of intention is best described and used herein as a *sankalpa*, a Sanskrit word that implies seeking the highest truth. A sankalpa turns the heart inward. It is not driven by the ego to determine an aim or measurable goal. A sankalpa bubbles up from deeply listening to your most heartfelt desire. Invite in this deep listening. Nourish a calm abiding for your sankalpa to become clear. Breathe in its living message calling from within. Embrace its calling with deep trust. Though it may take a few days or even weeks, once your sankalpa takes form, it is expressed as a short, affirmative statement. The following are a few examples. I thrive in good health. I am present in all I do. Mental clarity guides my day. Joy abides in me. Ease flows through my pores and in all I do. I embody loving presence.

Once you have your sankalpa, and you may have more than one, hold your sankalpa fervently and actively in your heart and mind. You can silently repeat it three times with the open invitation to repeat it to yourself, like a mantra, throughout your waking hours and in your dreams. Another all-important aspect of a sankalpa is to believe that it, in fact, will manifest: that the force of the energy behind your sankalpa has been firmly planted in the firmament and its unfolding revelations will come into being. When mindfully microdosing, a magical alchemy between you, your sankalpa, and the mushrooms is ever possible. What actually gets revealed is left up to an abiding trust that your heartfelt desire has been embraced. Believe it will come into manifestation in all its perfection.

Unlike a packet of flower seeds, for example daisies, which you would plant in the garden with the specific intention to grow and bloom, a sankalpa's alchemy mimics the biology of the mushroom. The spore's nature is to instantaneously project outward, traveling in the air in all directions. Once it lands, mycelium forms and begins to grow its networks underground. These networks also expand in all directions, nourishing an astonishing array of life. Some give rise to plant life that reveals itself above the surface, before your very eyes—including the daisies in the garden. This unseen, interwoven web, started from spores, is actively creating and mutually supporting gifts of abundant life in all its forms. Your sankalpa can do the same. So let its energy be received and taken like the mushroom spore: into open space and then to take root in unseen ways revealing bountiful gifts that enhance your life, nourish wholeness and well-being, and grow greater interconnectedness to all life. In this way, your sankalpa becomes your guiding intention. I invite you to look at these unfolding revelations as a magical garden, one that you have started from a deep sense of your own heartfelt desire.

During your journey, you will most likely notice benefits as well as face some challenges. Some things will take root right away, while others decay and wilt away. Perhaps some challenges, such as health, relationships, or work-related issues, like weeds, lessen and may even start to be overtaken with daisies. However, some challenges may initially seem amplified though your clarity to understand them may deepen. Just like after a summer's rain, more weeds may come to the surface but the soft moist soil makes their removal almost effortless. Your garden's growth is not a linear, step-by-step process. It is an ever-changing phenomena of coming into being, ripening, and dispersing into other ways of being. This nature of impermanence can be held in awe and wonder. Likewise, revel in the way your unique journey will unfold. Hold the benefits like blossoming gifts in wonder, while letting go of others with grace. All transforms into the beauty that is your life. Let your intention be the alchemy, or magic, if you will, between you and the mushrooms in your journey ahead.

Be sure to place your intention, written in a short sentence, into the Preparation section of the journal. The intention may change as the journey proceeds, so feel free to edit or rewrite any new intentions. You may want to write them in the spores scattered throughout the journal. In this way, your intentions are gentle whispers from your heart, and reminders of the magical alchemy of their manifestation. As part of their inherent intelligence, spores grow thread-like branches, called hyphae, in all directions; this is illustrated in the growing mycelial network found throughout the journal. You may want to add guiding messages, insights, or fill out each growing network with colors, words, or other creative inspirations. How they express themselves are part of the mystery of infinite possibilities and can find expression in the journal. Whatever you decide, the invitation is to co-create your own unique mindful microdosing journal in a way that is meaningful to you.

Journey — Active Microdosing

Microdosing is not a singular profound journey as it can be with macrodosing, but it can still yield profound effects and benefits both immediately and over time. Therefore, the period of active microdosing can be thought of as a journey. This section of the journal gives expression to observations, deep insights, ah-ha moments, changes of perspective, benefits, and challenges, and other areas you choose to focus in on. It holds space for what arises in your heart and mind without judgment, and in so doing further nourishes your experience.

As you start actively microdosing, you may want to bring heightened attention to the nuts and bolts of the journey itself. Though information on dosing, calibrating, and protocol is readily available on the web, having a coach or guide or joining a group at this stage can be most helpful. In fact, it can be the determining factor in supporting a more mindfulness-based approach to microdosing. Ten percent of a recreational dose is commonly considered a microdose, but 2.5%-12.5% is a wider margin also used as a range. There are many people of different sensitivities, conditions, and constitutions that dose far below that figure to ensure they are below a threshold, as described by Fadiman; while others may need slightly more. Most common is to start with a low minimum effective dose and work your way up in slow increments. A coach or guide, either on an individual basis or within a group setting can help you determine yours. It is recommended to keep a keen eye on dosage, time of day, and protocol until you find your sweet spot, especially when microdosing for the first time. Eventually, rather than a pre-determined, fixed amount, a more fluid process may unfold: your sweet spot becoming more like a sweet zone. What is right for one person at any given time and in different circumstances tends to be unique to that person. Your cycle may last approximately six weeks, as is common, but can be up to a few months. However long it is, a break between cycles of two to four-weeks or even several months is recommended. A microdosing motto, "Start low, go slow, and take time off," seems worthy of heeding. You may want to use a few pages of the journal to note and organize this information in a way that is helpful to you. In the end, approaching microdosing from a purely linear framework can be limiting, but it may be a judicious way to start. Over time, a more fluid, heart-centered journey emerges. As your relationship grows with the mushrooms, so, too, does intuitive knowing guide you.

Sitting down for a mindfulness practice, but before inviting in that first breath with full awareness, there is space for making a transition from daily life to an inner practice. So, too, with microdosing. This moment arises upon ingesting the mushrooms. Invite your intention into present awareness. Repeat it silently. Embody the conviction that your intention and the mushrooms have an alchemy to be revealed and manifested. Then let go, and with trust, awareness, and equanimity, be present with whatever arises.

As the journey proceeds, and the days and weeks progress, you may find that some old habits or ways of thinking and being are no longer needed, and fresh perspectives emerge. While journaling, these may take the form of coloring in or adding to the drawing, or they may be in words, paragraphs, or other forms and shapes. You may have included weeds in the beginning and they become fewer and fewer in proceeding pages. Perhaps you add some seeds that are germinating, or new buds appearing, or flowers in full bloom. Maybe you color with more vibrant markers; or you choose to add sparkles, decals, or mementos. Whatever arises has its place here. Invite in a sense of playfulness as you create and observe.

Another area you may want to make space for is the possibility that the mushrooms may be expressing themselves through you. What are their messages? Is there a growing relationship between you and the mushrooms? Listen carefully, especially when connecting to your intention upon ingesting them. You may want to include an illustration, an acknowledgment, or expression of gratitude toward the mushrooms as a daily part of the journal.

Seeing the petals of a daisy through a magnifying glass allows a gardener to get a closer look and make more precise observations. In a similar way, having a lens or framework magnifies observations you make in your own microdosing journey, lending greater inquiry and deeper reflection. This kind of self-inquiry invites mindful awareness as an integral part of the microdosing journey.

A framework is meant to shed more light on what you are observing, and is never meant to limit the experience. However, a framework is a specific lens of focus so it naturally influences your observations. For instance, if the focus is physical health, then you will probably bring more acute observations to your physical health, and pay less attention to other aspects of your overall health. With this understanding, a common framework followed for microdosing is the lens of the four dimensions of well-being: physical, emotional, cognitive, and spiritual. This is similar to many traditional ways of knowing that consider four aspects of being: body, mind, emotion, and spirit. A yogic perspective observes experience through the lens of five sheaths: physical, energetic, mental, wisdom, and bliss. A Buddhist approach, also used in Tibetan medicine for overall health, considers the five elements of earth, water, fire, air, and space. Three facets found in Buddhism, thought, word, and deed, can also be used as a framework. Or, you may want to look at your behavior, attitudes, and moods. You may want to try using different frameworks during different cycles of microdosing, and you may want to compare a cycle without using a framework at all. Whichever framework you choose, if you note it down in Preparation, it can serve as a powerful point of comparison. Then you can use the same lens of inquiry in the Journey and Integration sections. Additionally, a framework can be especially helpful when calibrating to find your sweet spot.

No matter how you approach your journey, enhanced well-being can be considered beyond the physical, beyond the seen and measurable. Some of the frameworks presented above capture this understanding by including categories such as spiritual, spirit, or bliss. This ephemeral inner knowing of your own well-being can be placed front and center of your experience if you so choose. Another aspect is your living connection with the natural world. Inspiration from the Mayans includes being in equilibrium with nature as an actual part of what it means to be healthy. Can you see ways in which microdosing enriches this relationship for your own health?

The unseen mycelial network, given healthy conditions, nourishes from beneath the forest floor. It directs nutrients in ways that are mutually beneficial for healthy growth above and below. This reciprocity alights a deep-seated impulse of mutual support. Attune to this symbiotic relationship in yourself to observe the ways you, too, nourish and support what you feel deeply connected to. It may be in kinder words you speak when engaging with family, friends, or others. As in this example, reciprocity is not just in thought, but it is also in word and deed. It may be those words spoken with greater kindness, or making a warm meal for your elderly neighbor, or contributing time to support your community. Sacred reciprocity has no bounds. What reciprocal relationships are becoming stronger in your life? How do you support more flourishing?

The concept of sacred reciprocity is seen most clearly with the natural world. It speaks to each individual's relationship to ecological restoration. How is this showing up in your relationship with the natural world? As you feel a growing connection to the natural world, so too can mutual flourishing strengthen. In what ways is this expressing itself through you? It may be by planting a native tree, joining a group that helps the environment, or funding a campaign. Quieter ways may be equally powerful: sitting under a tree and speaking to it, perhaps burying a poem beneath its roots, or ensuring its healthy growth and that of its immediate environment. Sacred reciprocity and mutual flourishing may be at the heart of ensuring harmonious balance.

Integration — Self-reflection and Transformation

This section captures how the microdosing journey has now become a living expression in you. Who are you becoming? Where has your heart led you? In what ways are you offering gifts to others? Sitting in calm abiding before ending a mindfulness practice offers a precious space in time to feel a more embodied presence, a greater sense of wholeness and well-being. This gathering of what has arisen is a pause before transitioning from inner to outer activity. It can serve as a daily reminder to integrate more mindfulness into daily life.

After several weeks of microdosing, there is also a pause, a break from microdosing, before another cycle begins. This resting period offers a time to acknowledge and embody the bountiful gifts of your microdosing journey and contemplate their meaningful, active integration into your life. Many of these gifts can be seen, yet many, like the mycelial network itself, may not seem so apparent. However, like this underground network, connections grow and neural pathways continue to fire as long as you nourish their growth. Actively paying attention, actively choosing habits of mind, actively reconnecting, remembering, and embodying behaviors that stimulate this growth in healthy ways will bring flourishing to your magical garden. Conversely, what may have diminished, those ways of being that don't serve you, can naturally release. When whispered away with gratitude, they turn into manna for growth. They can be thought of as needed decay, churning into essential nutrients to nourish the very networks that fuel new life. These networks manifest in a multitude of ways: a plethora of flowers blooming, butterflies now returning to their long-lost habitat, fruits ripening, and saplings seeking light. There is a restoring of the ecological landscape of more balance and harmony. Transformation is always possible. What was magic is now manifest. This inner garden of your essential nature evolves into an enchanted forest garden, a sanctuary protected by strong and sturdy growth.

The drawings of the magical gardens in the Preparation and Journey sections have transformed into an enchanted forest garden in Integration. Color in your sanctuary, including the sturdy oak tree representing wisdom and protection. The nearby saplings of new growth may evoke new beginnings, rebirth, a freshness in perspectives and focus. Their innate strength and resilience are coming into being, needing healthy conditions to survive and grow. What has come to life in your enchanted forest garden sanctuary? What unexpected magic now appears? What is still growing into fullness? What stands strong? What beauty and joy are now soaring? Pay attention to growth below the surface as well as above. What may lie dormant? What has decayed? What new growth needs special nurturing to survive and flourish?

Gratitude, like air, is an unseen force moving through everything. In the following pages, you may want to draw a harvest basket with your own cornucopia of gratitudes and fill it in ways that illustrate what you cherish. Use beautiful colors, markers, or paints to celebrate this harvest.

Like a mushroom's constitution, you, too, are composed mainly of water. You may notice that this life-giving element appears in the enchanted forest garden. Water flows into a pond, creating a well-spring of nourishing qualities where a lotus flower is in full bloom. The lotus is an inspiring example of the inherent ability to grow from the deepest darkness, mired in muck, reach for the light, and eventually transform into its full potential. How are you reaching for the light? In what ways are you transforming? A stream, coming from beyond the forest grove, feeds the pond. What is cascading in your life to bring self-nourishment? Can you dip into its waters for strength, peace, and other qualities of well-being that feel healing and bring more wholeness? Once nourished, what is the ripple effect? How do you bring these elements into your life? What concrete actions are you taking? What has become more fluid? How have any courses or currents of your flow changed?

Metaphors and illustrations are creative ways to express feelings and emotions of less linear, non-ordinary states of mind. Recapturing these feelings and emotions in embodied and somatic expression can also keep them alive. So part of integration is finding ways to reconnect, remember, and evoke these ways of being. Forest walks, mindfulness practices, breathwork, movement, gardening, drawing, painting, sound healing, cooking, clay work, and other creative expressions can enhance and deepen these connections. Woven into these practices is the force of gratitude in the form of thanksgiving, prayer, mindfulness, poetry, or daily journaling. You may want to use this journal to jot down ideas, ambitions, or reflections as you engage in these and other activities that support your integration.

The Integration section of the journal is an open invitation to express all that is in your heart and mind—to celebrate all of whom you have become and are becoming. The following prompts are offered for self-reflection on your own deepening understanding. What fresh perspectives or new awarenesses do you have? What is different in your life? Has anything unintended arisen? What of your social connections? And your connections to nature? Do you feel healthier? How? Is there a greater sense of wholeness? How is it embodied?

Integration is a continuous process of becoming, dissolving, and coming into being throughout every part of the journey and every moment in time. Like any cycle of life, and like the mushrooms themselves, there is no beginning or end point. Integration may include looking back at the Preparation pages and reviewing where you started and any intentions you noted. How does that resonate now? What has been integrated? What is still to manifest? How has your story changed? Where is your heart leading you now?

After these contemplations, you may want to write a letter to yourself. Or you may want to write a letter to the mushrooms in gratitude and acknowledgment for what they have brought to your journey. An additional possibility is for the mushrooms to be the author penning an epistle to you. What deep wisdom has come from their offerings out to you? What kind of relationship are you developing with them?

In the days, weeks, or months ahead, you may want to revisit and add more to your journal, or start a new one. As you fill the pages of this journal with mindful awareness and on-going integration, I hope what gets expressed seeps into your very being, growing ever-expanding connections like the mycelial network itself. I hope that it optimizes your well-being and brings greater connection to your own ever-existing wholeness and to the greater whole of which you are always a part. I hope this journey of mindful microdosing cultivates a spaciousness of mind and an expansiveness of heart in the all-knowing present moment. For in that stillness there emerges a sacred connection to all.

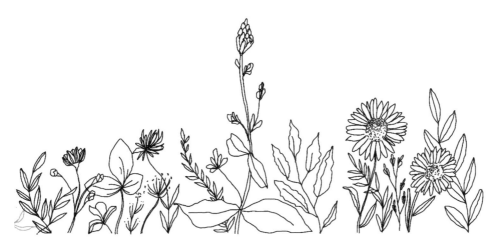

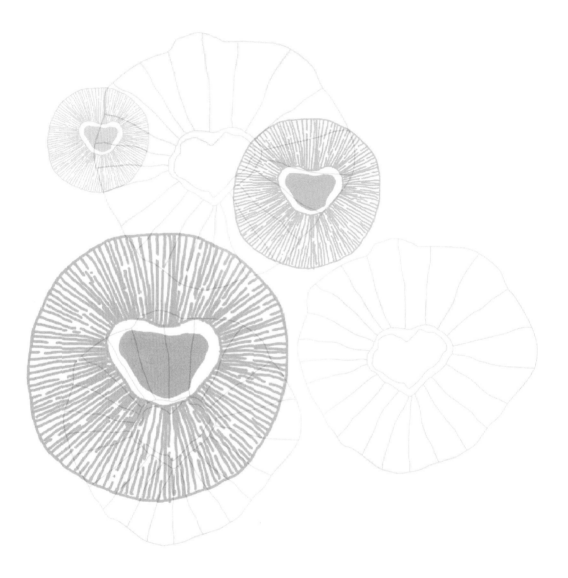

PREPARATION

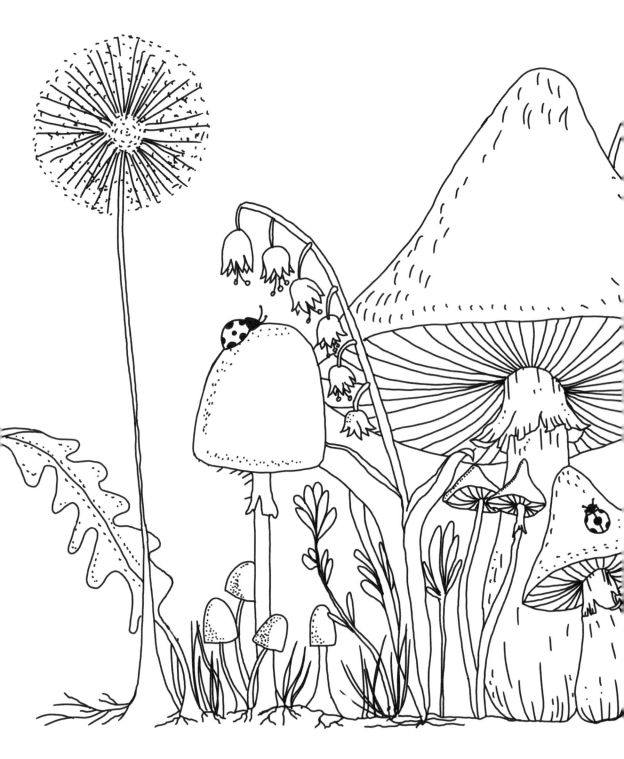

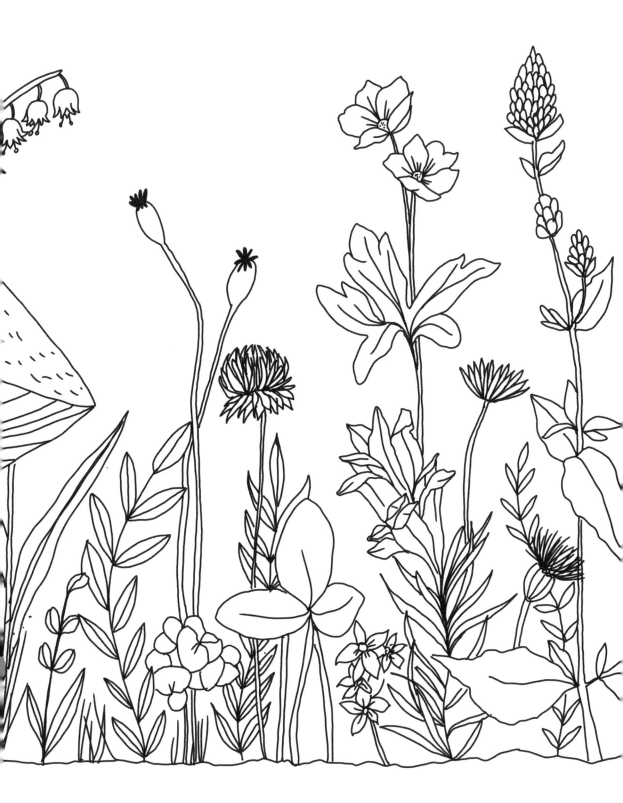

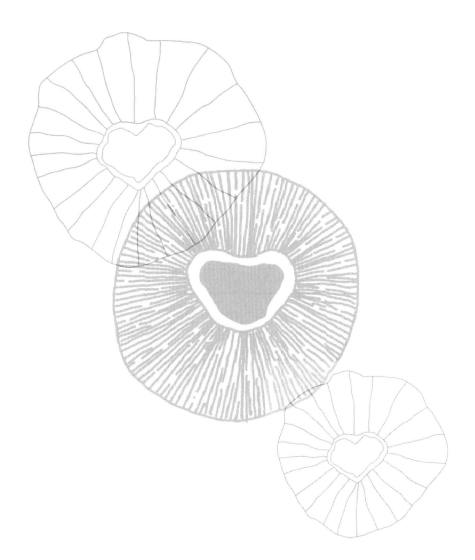

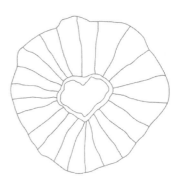

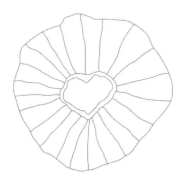

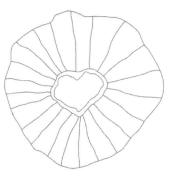

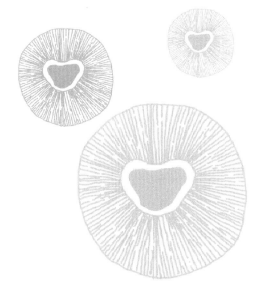

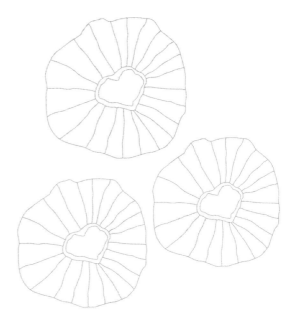

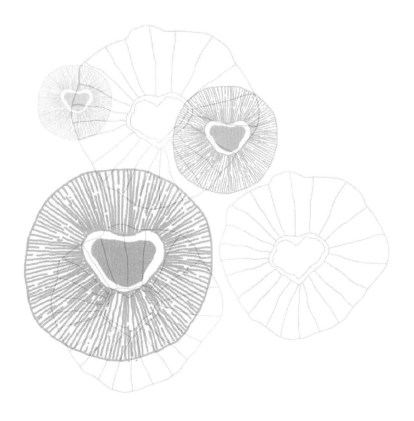

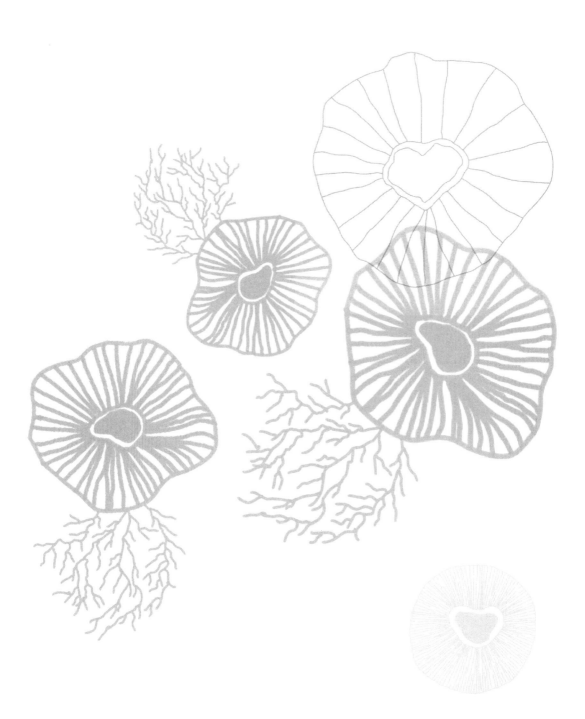

JOURNEY

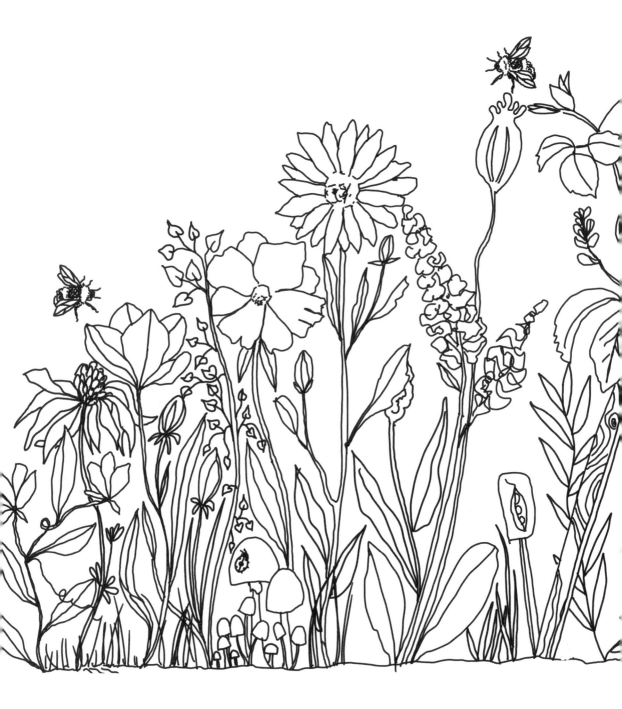

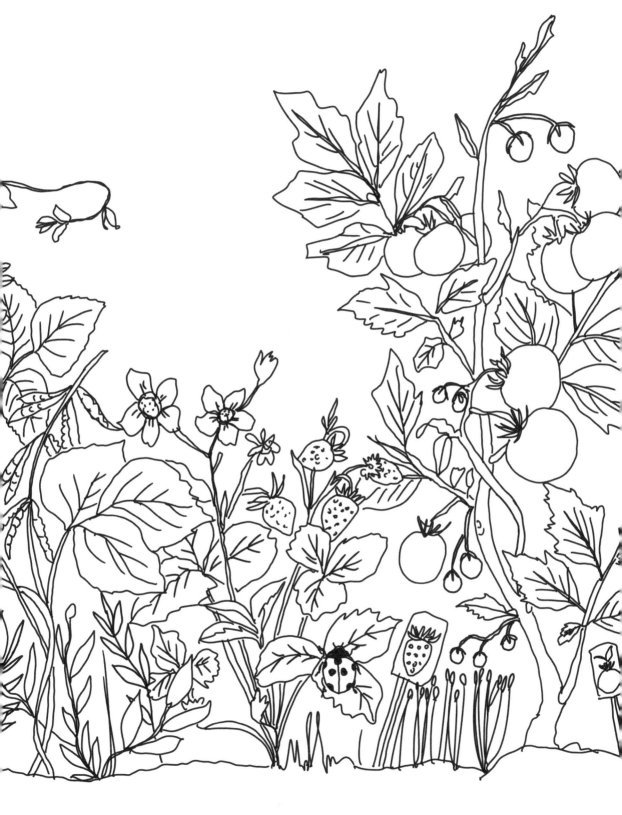

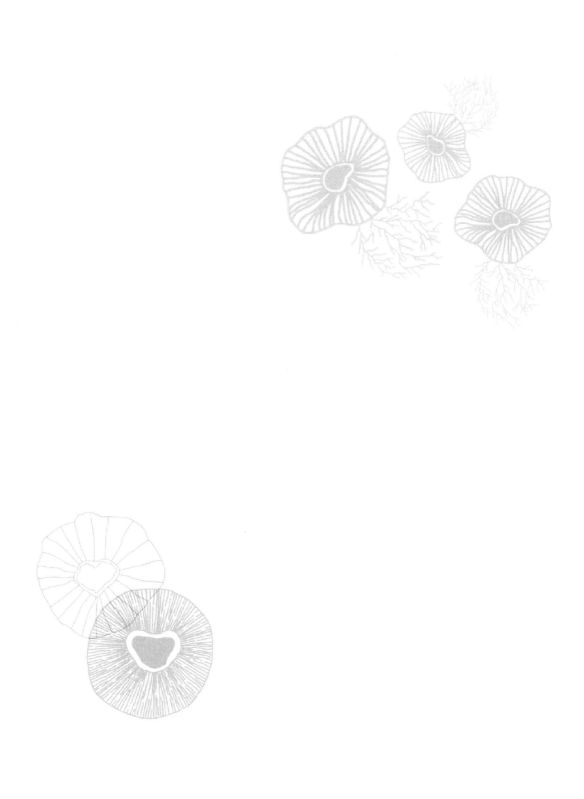

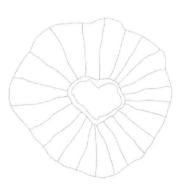

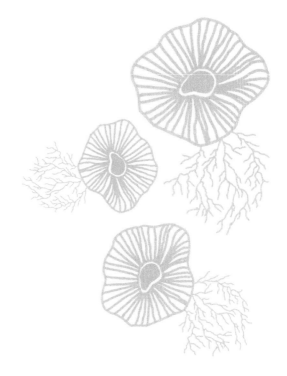

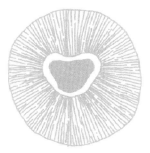

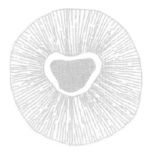

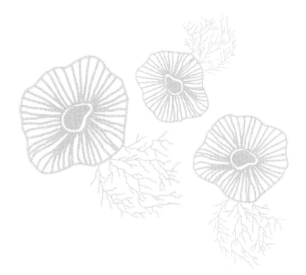

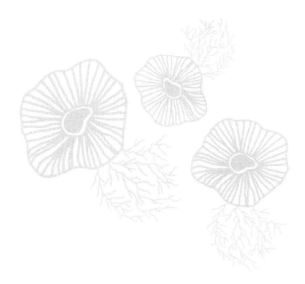
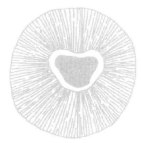

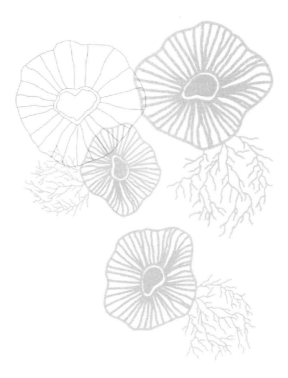

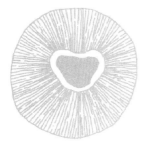

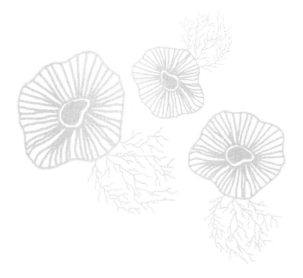

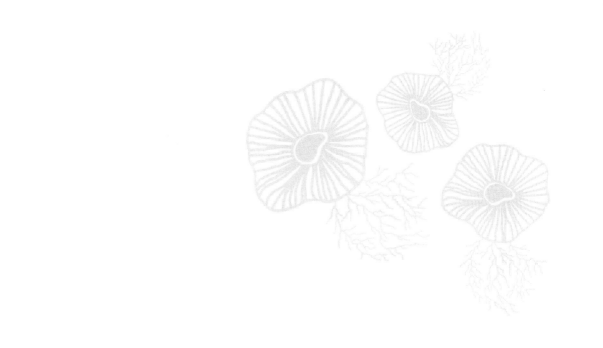

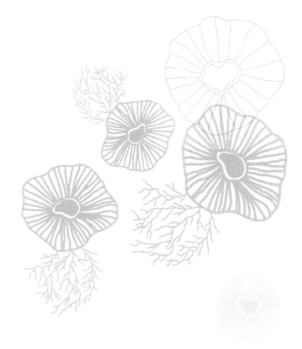

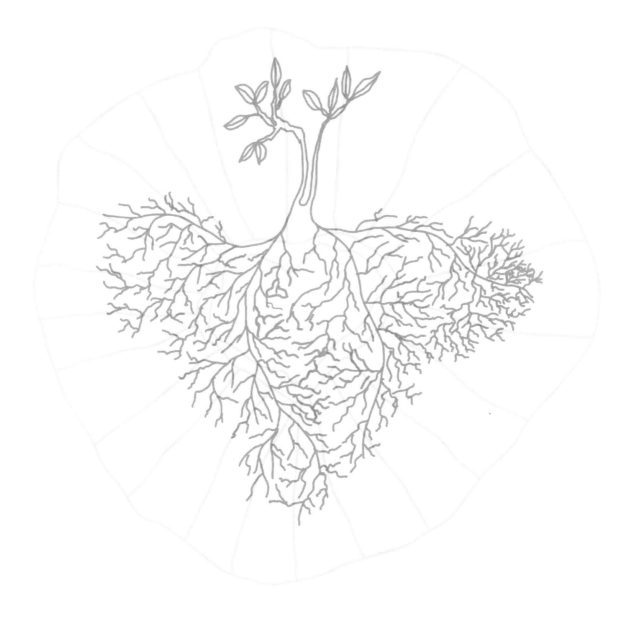

INTEGRATION

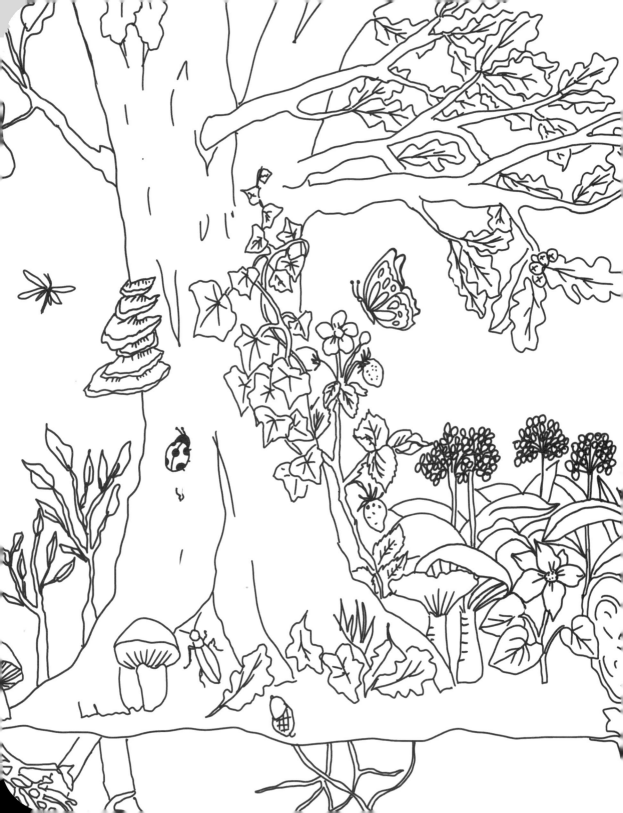

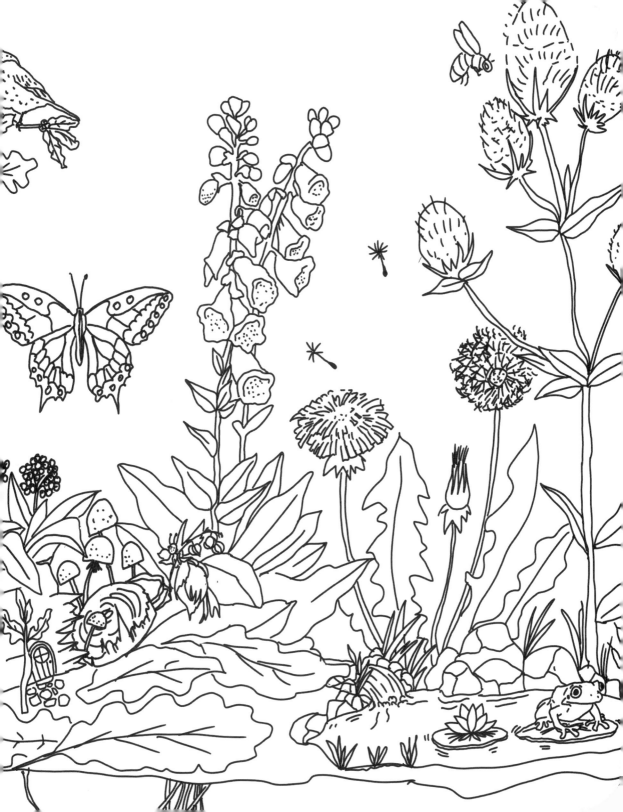

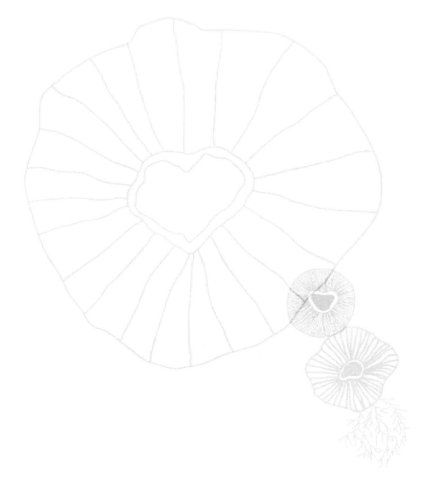

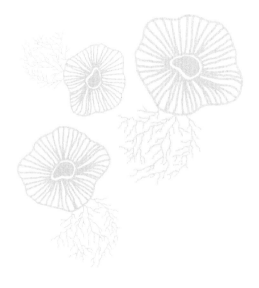

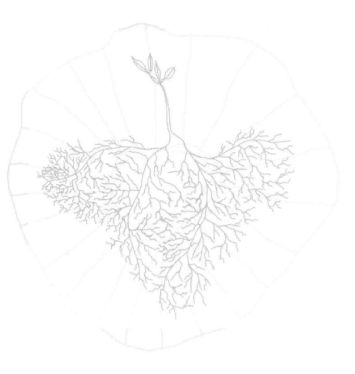

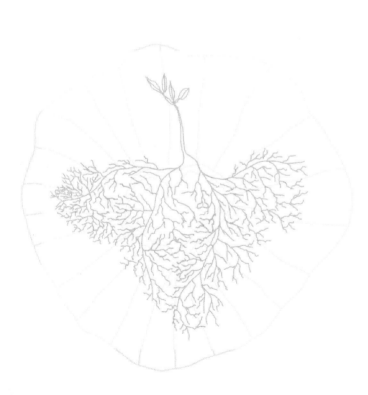

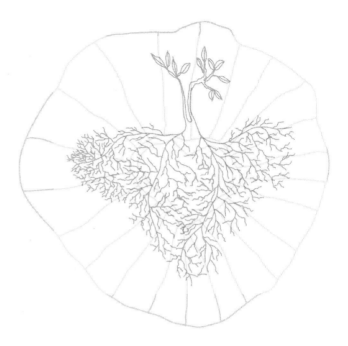

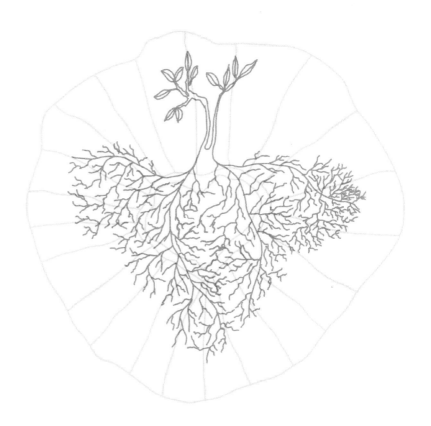

MORE INVITATIONS

Mindful microdosing is built on the understanding of your mindful awareness and discernment to ensure a safe foundation to explore. A more mindfulness-based approach to first-time microdosing usually includes a coach or joining a group for guidance and support; likewise, certain medical, physical, or mental health considerations are contraindicated* or are best supported by a team that may include a medical doctor, psychiatrist, or other professional. The information below is for educational purposes only and does not substitute professional medical advice or consultation with healthcare professionals. While the information does not condone or promote illegal activity, the information supplied is in recognition of the need for on-going educational information, harm reduction, and to contribute to a narrative that supports mindful microdosing. Mindfulness aims to balance heart and mind; it can become a dance rather than a linear, step-by-step process, but it helps to know the initial steps when first learning a new dance.

CHOOSING YOUR ALLY Dosing Ranges For Some Commonly Used Microdosing Substances*

People of different ages, sensitivities, conditions, and constitutions dose at the lower range or even lower. Consider your choice of substance, or ally, as each has its own unique signature personality.
Mindful Inquiry: Which substance or ally and what amount best match my intention?

Substance	Average Microdosing Range
Dried Psilocybin Mushrooms	0.05g (50 mg) – 0.25g (250 mg)
LSD, ICP-LSD, IP-LSD	2.5mcg – 12.5mcg
Dried San Pedro Cactus	0.025g
Whole B. Caapi Vine	2.5g – 10g

ESTABLISHING EASE A Microdosing Calibration Schedule To Find Your Sweet Spot *

The process of learning about what is right for you and feeling completely safe in that process establishes ease. You may even want to start at a lower first dose to begin calibration. Likewise, lower calibration increments can be followed throughout the process. In addition, another calibration dose or more may be needed to complete your process. Once you do find your sweet spot, there is no need to increase your dose. Then follow one of the protocols found on the next page.
Mindful Inquiry: What is my lowest calibration dose #1 to ease into actively microdosing?

Finding your minimum effective dose	Dried Psilocybin Mushrooms	LSD, ICP-LSD, IP-LSD	Dried San Pedro Cactus	Whole B. Caapi Vine
Calibration Dose #1	0.05g (50 mg)	2.5 mcg	0.05g / 50 mg	2.5g
Calibration Dose #2	0.10g / 100 mg	5 mcg	0.10g / 100 mg	3.75g
Calibration Dose #3	0.15g / 150 mg	7.5 mcg	0.15g / 150 mg	5g
Calibration Dose #4	0.20g / 200 mg	10 mcg	0.20g / 200 mg	7.5g

*See: https://microdosinginstitute.com/ The Microdosing Institute, for information on contraindications, coaching, and programs. Modified charts are used with permission from The Microdosing Institute, The Netherlands.

TAKING FIRST STEPS Microdosing Calibration Tracker

A common first step for those new to microdosing is to track the calibration process. Not surprisingly, seasoned microdosers commonly find their sweet spot is lower when approaching microdosing with a mindfulness-based lens. The chart is designed for you to use as best fits your needs, if at all. You can note the date or day of the week and then include exact dose, time of day, and other information such as mushroom strain or source. Dosing is usually done on alternate days but it is common that this does not happen due to personal circumstances. Keep in mind that you may find your sweet spot after the first calibration which is why only that dose has a number. Add the number to each calibration dose you need, adding more doses if needed.

Mindful Inquiry: What are my first steps? What notations are helpful? What are some observations?

dose #1				
dose				
dose				
dose				
dose				

FINDING YOUR RHYTHM Common Protocols for A Microdosing Cycle

Below are different ways to dose, or protocols that are common, to help you find a rhythm that feels right for you. Once you have your sweet spot, typically one protocol is followed for a 6–8 week cycle. Then follows a break or resting period of 2–4 weeks or up to several months.

A microdosing motto: Start low, go slow, and take time off.

Mindful Inquiry: What rhythm best supports my intention?

	M	T	W	T	F	S	S
Microdosing Institute Protocol	M	T	W	T	F	S	S
		1 DAY ON, 1 DAY OFF					
"Fadiman" Protocol	M	T	W	T	F	S	S
		1 DAY ON, 2 DAYS OFF					
"Stamets" Protocol	M	T	W	T	F	S	S
		4 DAYS ON, 3 DAYS OFF					
Work Week Protocol	M	T	W	T	F	S	S
		5 DAYS ON, 2 DAYS OFF					
Intuitive Protocol	M	T	W	T	F	S	S
		USUALLY AFTER SEVERAL CYCLES, FOLLOW YOUR OWN INTUITION					

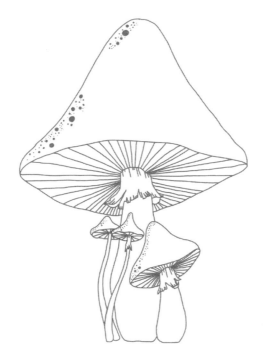

ABOUT THE AUTHOR & ILLUSTRATOR

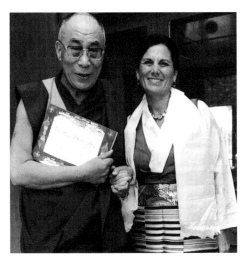

Lauren Alderfer is the award-winning mindfulness author of *Teaching from the Heart of Mindfulness*. She also wrote the popular children's book, *Mindful Monkey, Happy Panda* as well as other Buddhist stories. Leaving the U.S. to start her career in Ecuador, Lauren lived in the Andean region for over twenty years. She then lived on the Indian subcontinent for nearly two more decades. There, Lauren was immersed in language preservation in the Tibetan refugee community. This journal weaves together her lived experiences to give a unique voice to mindful microdosing. Lauren is a certified Microdosing Coach and holds a PhD in Global Education Leadership. Visit www.laurenalderfer.com

Mexican artist **Mariana Juarez (MJ)** has been painting since she was five years old. She feels Mother Nature calls her to explore and create. Indeed, MJ's fanciful botanical art offers a magnifying glass to the natural world, plants and animals being her favorite motifs. MJ's coloring books bring out creativity in children and adults alike. She also paints bold, colorful murals. Her work can be seen on the façades of colonial homes throughout San Miguel de Allende where she lives with her wife, Kathryn, and cat, Lucy. MJ studied Visual Arts at Bellas Artes, Morelia. Visit www.mjmuralart.com

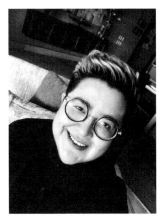